Worksheets for Cognitive Behavioral Therapy for Bipolar Disorder

CBT Workbook to Deal with Stress, Anxiety, Anger, Control Mood, Learn New Behaviors & Regulate Emotions

Portia Cruise

© 2019 Portia Cruise

All rights reserved.

This book or any portion thereof may not be reproduced or used in any manner whatsoever without the express written permission of the publisher except for the use of brief quotations in a book review.

You are welcome to join the Fan's Corner, here

Disclaimer

The advice and strategies found within may not be suitable for every situation. This work is sold with the understanding that neither the author nor the publisher is held responsible for the results accrued from the advice in this book.

About the Worksheet

Congratulations on getting this CBT workbook. You can monitor the progress of your therapy using Cognitive Behavioral Therapy with this logbook and record the thoughts you have for different situations.

A CBT worksheet (also called a thought record) can help you think about your thinking. It is an essential tool for cognitive therapy that contains a series of questions aimed at guiding you step-by-step through the process of identifying your negative thinking and changing it.

It can be used by those who suffer from many mental health challenges that include but not limited to insomnia, borderline personality disorder, obsessive-compulsive disorder (OCD) psychosis, anxiety, bipolar disorder, eating disorders - such as anorexia and bulimia, phobias, schizophrenia, depression, panic disorder, alcohol misuse and post-traumatic stress disorder (PTSD)

Experience has shown that it is better to enter the details of your activity into the logbook as soon as is possible when the information is still fresh in your memory.

This logbook is more than just a record of your thought records, it also covers your action plans and possible improvement you plan to undertake.

Worksheets for Cognitive Behavioral Therapy is a reliable partner in your journey to get the best out of your Therapeutic sessions.

Good Luck in your healing process!!!

Personal Details

Name:	
Age:	
Diagnosed Issue	
Address:	
City:	
Phone Number:	
Emergency Contact Number:	
Mental Health Institute	
Dr. in Charge	

Personal Goals

Objective of Therapy

_____

_____

_____

_____

Define Milestones

_____

_____

_____

_____

Define Motivation

_____

_____

_____

_____

Decide Target Date

_____

_____

How to Use This Worksheet

This worksheet may be used under the guidance of an appropriate health professional.

The first three steps typically help you to correctly identify the essential things you need to change and should be used as motivation.

1. The situation

This important step is used to briefly describe the specific situation that led to your unpleasant feelings. It is designed to ensure you do not forget the situation when you later review your notes.

Example: At a social event today, I said something that I believe was inappropriate. I felt embarrassed and later I felt anxious thinking about it.

2. Initial thought

This next step is used to describe the first thoughts that entered your mind as a result of the situation. It could well be a subconscious response of thoughts of something you have previously had.

Example: I feel like a miserable failure. I am anxious people will judge me. I hate having this distinct feeling of making foolish mistakes.

3. Thought Consequences

You implement this step to identify why you want this way of thinking changed and what the possible consequences are if you do not change. Here you determine what the physical, professional, psychological, and relationship consequences are.

Example: If I do not stop this inappropriate way of thinking and beating up myself, I could become miserable. My negativity could equally affect my health and my relationships. Unless I stop believing I am an imminent failure, I could end up losing my self-respect and start behaving like a real failure.

These next 3 steps (4-6) typically help you realize your negative thoughts do not have any facts supporting them, but are instead driven by certain false beliefs that you acquired while growing up.

4. Challenge Your Initial Thought

In this step, you challenge yourself to objectively determine if this specific way of thinking has ever been beneficial to you in the past. Here you correctly determine the specific facts that challenge or support your initial thought and dig out your personal strength you may have undoubtedly overlooked. If someone else was in such a situation, what possible advice would you offer the person?

Example: When I intentionally try to be perfect, I feel I am too hard on myself which invariably makes me feel overwhelmed. I reckon I really do not have to be perfect, after all, most people who constantly beat themselves up end up being insecure and nervous compared to those who are easy on themselves and take things in their stride. Mistakes are a part of life and not sure a big deal.

5. Negative thinking

You can use this column to summarize the kind of negative thinking that triggered your initial thought. You use this opportunity to carefully identify one or more of the basic types of negative thinking: should-statements, mind-reading, catastrophizing, focusing on the negatives, negative self-labeling, all-or-nothing.

Example: I was focusing on just the negatives and believed nothing good could come out of my situation. I was catastrophizing.

6. Background

This step is an optional one, but very useful in trying to identify the root cause of your thoughts. You achieve this by going back in time to when you first started having this kind of thought as the first thought that comes to your mind when faced with such situations so that you can identify how deep the roots go. You also try to remember anyone else you know who also reasons this way. You do this so that you determine how much effect this has had on you.

Example: I still regularly hear the familiar voice of my parents saying I'll never amount to anything.

You use the next 2 steps (7-8) to come up with more positive ways of thinking and come up with great positive affirmations to lift up yourself.

7. Alternative thinking

Now that you are beginning to understand your negative thinking better, it is time to determine how if given another chance you could have handled the situation better by removing all the negative assumptions and instead think of positive facts or possibilities that you may have ignored.

> Example: I only just have to strive to be better at what I do and do not have to be perfect since no one really is. I undoubtedly possess unique strengths that countless others can appreciate. I notice I always feel better when I am kind to myself and will do well to get rid of this negative thinking.

8. Positive belief and affirmation

Now is the time to take steps to begin healing. Jot down various affirmations aimed at forming a positive image of yourself, to reflect a more improved healthy approach to life that you can use also use as a future reference.

> Example: I am an amazing person with lots of strength and positive vibes.

The next two steps (9-10) can help you use the new thinking you have naturally acquired from the previous steps to make your life better.

9. Action plan

The essence of this next step is to take advantage of your increased awareness and determine how you plan to act if this situation comes up again so that you can learn the best ways to overcome your natural tendencies and be better equipped to deal with the situation. Think of all the extraordinary strengths you have relating to the situation and write them down. Work out how to deal with triggers that make you want to go back to your old habits.

> Example: Anytime I am going to a social setting, I will subtly remind myself that being hard on myself does me no good and in situations where I invariably make mistakes, I will try not to dwell on the negatives by reminding myself of my previous success in similar circumstances. I will be kind first to myself and then others.

10. Improvement

This key step is used to positively reinforce the fundamental idea that voluntarily changing your thinking, can change your life. You utilize this to tell yourself of the need to progressively improve and be generally optimistic about what life offers.

Every time you fill a thought record, you will naturally begin to notice after a while that certain things keep recurring as part of initial thoughts and the chain of events that happen after that. You will also find it is becoming easier for you to identify your negative thoughts and come up with alternatives that better for you.

Worksheets for Cognitive Behavioral Therapy

Date: ___/___/_____

Situation	
Initial Thought	
Thought Consequences	
Challenge your Initial Thought	
Negative Thinking	
Background	
Alternative Thinking	
Positive Belief and Affirmation	
Action Plan	
Improvement	

Dr's Notes: _____

_____

Name: _____ Date: _____ Sign: _____

© 2019 Portia Cruise. *Cognitive Behavioral Therapy Worksheets.* **Copyrighted Material**

Worksheets for Cognitive Behavioral Therapy

Date: ____/____/_____

Situation	
Initial Thought	
Thought Consequences	
Challenge your Initial Thought	
Negative Thinking	
Background	
Alternative Thinking	
Positive Belief and Affirmation	
Action Plan	
Improvement	

Dr's Notes: _____

_____

Name: _____ Date: _____ Sign: _____

© 2019 Portia Cruise. *Cognitive Behavioral Therapy Worksheets.* **Copyrighted Material**

Worksheets for Cognitive Behavioral Therapy

Date: ___/___/_____

Situation	
Initial Thought	
Thought Consequences	
Challenge your Initial Thought	
Negative Thinking	
Background	
Alternative Thinking	
Positive Belief and Affirmation	
Action Plan	
Improvement	

Dr's Notes: _____

_____

Name: _____ Date: _____ Sign: _____

© 2019 Portia Cruise. *Cognitive Behavioral Therapy Worksheets.* **Copyrighted Material**

Worksheets for Cognitive Behavioral Therapy

Date: ____/____/_____

Situation	
Initial Thought	
Thought Consequences	
Challenge your Initial Thought	
Negative Thinking	
Background	
Alternative Thinking	
Positive Belief and Affirmation	
Action Plan	
Improvement	

Dr's Notes: _____

_____

Name: _____ Date: _____ Sign: _____

© 2019 Portia Cruise. *Cognitive Behavioral Therapy Worksheets.* **Copyrighted Material**

Worksheets for Cognitive Behavioral Therapy

Date: ____/____/_____

Situation	
Initial Thought	
Thought Consequences	
Challenge your Initial Thought	
Negative Thinking	
Background	
Alternative Thinking	
Positive Belief and Affirmation	
Action Plan	
Improvement	

Dr's Notes: _____

_____

Name: _____   Date: _____   Sign: _____

© 2019 Portia Cruise. *Cognitive Behavioral Therapy Worksheets.* **Copyrighted Material**

Worksheets for Cognitive Behavioral Therapy

Date: ___/___/_____

Situation	
Initial Thought	
Thought Consequences	
Challenge your Initial Thought	
Negative Thinking	
Background	
Alternative Thinking	
Positive Belief and Affirmation	
Action Plan	
Improvement	

Dr's Notes: _____

_____

Name: _____ Date: _____ Sign: _____

© 2019 Portia Cruise. *Cognitive Behavioral Therapy Worksheets.* **Copyrighted Material**

Worksheets for Cognitive Behavioral Therapy

Date: ____/____/_____

Situation	
Initial Thought	
Thought Consequences	
Challenge your Initial Thought	
Negative Thinking	
Background	
Alternative Thinking	
Positive Belief and Affirmation	
Action Plan	
Improvement	

Dr's Notes: _____

_____

Name: _____ Date: _____ Sign: _____

Worksheets for Cognitive Behavioral Therapy

Date: ___/___/_____

Situation	
Initial Thought	
Thought Consequences	
Challenge your Initial Thought	
Negative Thinking	
Background	
Alternative Thinking	
Positive Belief and Affirmation	
Action Plan	
Improvement	

Dr's Notes: _____

_____

Name: _____ Date: _____ Sign: _____

© 2019 Portia Cruise. *Cognitive Behavioral Therapy Worksheets.* Copyrighted Material

Worksheets for Cognitive Behavioral Therapy

Date: ___/___/_____

Situation	
Initial Thought	
Thought Consequences	
Challenge your Initial Thought	
Negative Thinking	
Background	
Alternative Thinking	
Positive Belief and Affirmation	
Action Plan	
Improvement	

Dr's Notes: _____

_____

Name: _____ Date: _____ Sign: _____

© 2019 Portia Cruise. *Cognitive Behavioral Therapy Worksheets.* Copyrighted Material

Worksheets for Cognitive Behavioral Therapy

Date: ____/____/_____

Situation	
Initial Thought	
Thought Consequences	
Challenge your Initial Thought	
Negative Thinking	
Background	
Alternative Thinking	
Positive Belief and Affirmation	
Action Plan	
Improvement	

Dr's Notes: _____

_____

Name: _____ Date: _____ Sign: _____

© 2019 Portia Cruise. *Cognitive Behavioral Therapy Worksheets.* **Copyrighted Material**

Worksheets for Cognitive Behavioral Therapy

Date: ___/___/_____

Situation	
Initial Thought	
Thought Consequences	
Challenge your Initial Thought	
Negative Thinking	
Background	
Alternative Thinking	
Positive Belief and Affirmation	
Action Plan	
Improvement	

Dr's Notes: _____

_____

Name: _____ Date: _____ Sign: _____

© 2019 Portia Cruise. *Cognitive Behavioral Therapy Worksheets.* **Copyrighted Material**

Worksheets for Cognitive Behavioral Therapy

Date: ____/____/_____

Situation	
Initial Thought	
Thought Consequences	
Challenge your Initial Thought	
Negative Thinking	
Background	
Alternative Thinking	
Positive Belief and Affirmation	
Action Plan	
Improvement	

Dr's Notes: _____

_____

Name: _____ Date: _____ Sign: _____

© 2019 Portia Cruise. *Cognitive Behavioral Therapy Worksheets.* **Copyrighted Material**

Worksheets for Cognitive Behavioral Therapy

Date: ____/____/_____

Situation	
Initial Thought	
Thought Consequences	
Challenge your Initial Thought	
Negative Thinking	
Background	
Alternative Thinking	
Positive Belief and Affirmation	
Action Plan	
Improvement	

Dr's Notes: _____

_____

Name: _____ Date: _____ Sign: _____

© 2019 Portia Cruise. *Cognitive Behavioral Therapy Worksheets.* Copyrighted Material

Worksheets for Cognitive Behavioral Therapy

Date: ____/____/_____

Situation	
Initial Thought	
Thought Consequences	
Challenge your Initial Thought	
Negative Thinking	
Background	
Alternative Thinking	
Positive Belief and Affirmation	
Action Plan	
Improvement	

Dr's Notes: _____

_____

Name: _____ Date: _____ Sign: _____

© 2019 Portia Cruise. *Cognitive Behavioral Therapy Worksheets.* **Copyrighted Material**

Worksheets for Cognitive Behavioral Therapy

Date: ___/___/_____

Situation	
Initial Thought	
Thought Consequences	
Challenge your Initial Thought	
Negative Thinking	
Background	
Alternative Thinking	
Positive Belief and Affirmation	
Action Plan	
Improvement	

Dr's Notes: _____

_____

Name: _____ Date: _____ Sign: _____

© 2019 Portia Cruise. *Cognitive Behavioral Therapy Worksheets.* **Copyrighted Material**

Worksheets for Cognitive Behavioral Therapy

Date: ___/___/_____

Situation	
Initial Thought	
Thought Consequences	
Challenge your Initial Thought	
Negative Thinking	
Background	
Alternative Thinking	
Positive Belief and Affirmation	
Action Plan	
Improvement	

Dr's Notes: _____

_____

Name: _____ Date: _____ Sign: _____

© 2019 Portia Cruise. *Cognitive Behavioral Therapy Worksheets.* Copyrighted Material

Worksheets for Cognitive Behavioral Therapy

Date: ___/___/_____

Situation	
Initial Thought	
Thought Consequences	
Challenge your Initial Thought	
Negative Thinking	
Background	
Alternative Thinking	
Positive Belief and Affirmation	
Action Plan	
Improvement	

Dr's Notes: _____

_____

Name: _____ Date: _____ Sign: _____

© 2019 Portia Cruise. *Cognitive Behavioral Therapy Worksheets.* Copyrighted Material

Worksheets for Cognitive Behavioral Therapy

Date: ____/____/_____

Situation	
Initial Thought	
Thought Consequences	
Challenge your Initial Thought	
Negative Thinking	
Background	
Alternative Thinking	
Positive Belief and Affirmation	
Action Plan	
Improvement	

Dr's Notes: _____

_____

Name: _____ Date: _____ Sign: _____

© 2019 Portia Cruise. *Cognitive Behavioral Therapy Worksheets.* Copyrighted Material

Worksheets for Cognitive Behavioral Therapy

Date: ____/____/_____

Situation	
Initial Thought	
Thought Consequences	
Challenge your Initial Thought	
Negative Thinking	
Background	
Alternative Thinking	
Positive Belief and Affirmation	
Action Plan	
Improvement	

Dr's Notes: _____

_____

Name: _____ Date: _____ Sign: _____

© 2019 Portia Cruise. *Cognitive Behavioral Therapy Worksheets.* Copyrighted Material

Worksheets for Cognitive Behavioral Therapy

Date: ___/___/_____

Situation	
Initial Thought	
Thought Consequences	
Challenge your Initial Thought	
Negative Thinking	
Background	
Alternative Thinking	
Positive Belief and Affirmation	
Action Plan	
Improvement	

Dr's Notes: _____

_____

Name: _____ Date: _____ Sign: _____

© 2019 Portia Cruise. *Cognitive Behavioral Therapy Worksheets.* Copyrighted Material

Worksheets for Cognitive Behavioral Therapy

Date: ___/___/_____

Situation	
Initial Thought	
Thought Consequences	
Challenge your Initial Thought	
Negative Thinking	
Background	
Alternative Thinking	
Positive Belief and Affirmation	
Action Plan	
Improvement	

Dr's Notes: _____

_____

Name: _____ Date: _____ Sign: _____

© 2019 Portia Cruise. *Cognitive Behavioral Therapy Worksheets.* **Copyrighted Material**

Worksheets for Cognitive Behavioral Therapy

Date: ____/____/_____

Situation	
Initial Thought	
Thought Consequences	
Challenge your Initial Thought	
Negative Thinking	
Background	
Alternative Thinking	
Positive Belief and Affirmation	
Action Plan	
Improvement	

Dr's Notes: _____

_____

Name: _____ Date: _____ Sign: _____

© 2019 Portia Cruise. *Cognitive Behavioral Therapy Worksheets.* Copyrighted Material

Worksheets for Cognitive Behavioral Therapy

Date: ____/____/_____

Situation	
Initial Thought	
Thought Consequences	
Challenge your Initial Thought	
Negative Thinking	
Background	
Alternative Thinking	
Positive Belief and Affirmation	
Action Plan	
Improvement	

Dr's Notes: _____

_____

Name: _____ Date: _____ Sign: _____

© 2019 Portia Cruise. *Cognitive Behavioral Therapy Worksheets.* Copyrighted Material

Worksheets for Cognitive Behavioral Therapy

Date: ____/____/_____

Situation	
Initial Thought	
Thought Consequences	
Challenge your Initial Thought	
Negative Thinking	
Background	
Alternative Thinking	
Positive Belief and Affirmation	
Action Plan	
Improvement	

Dr's Notes: _____

_____

Name: _____ Date: _____ Sign: _____

© 2019 Portia Cruise. *Cognitive Behavioral Therapy Worksheets.* **Copyrighted Material**

Worksheets for Cognitive Behavioral Therapy

Date: ____/____/_____

Situation	
Initial Thought	
Thought Consequences	
Challenge your Initial Thought	
Negative Thinking	
Background	
Alternative Thinking	
Positive Belief and Affirmation	
Action Plan	
Improvement	

Dr's Notes: _____

_____

Name: _____ Date: _____ Sign: _____

© 2019 Portia Cruise. *Cognitive Behavioral Therapy Worksheets.* **Copyrighted Material**

Worksheets for Cognitive Behavioral Therapy

Date: ____/____/_____

Situation	
Initial Thought	
Thought Consequences	
Challenge your Initial Thought	
Negative Thinking	
Background	
Alternative Thinking	
Positive Belief and Affirmation	
Action Plan	
Improvement	

Dr's Notes: _____

_____

Name: _____ Date: _____ Sign: _____

© 2019 Portia Cruise. *Cognitive Behavioral Therapy Worksheets.* **Copyrighted Material**

Worksheets for Cognitive Behavioral Therapy

Date: ____/____/_____

Situation	
Initial Thought	
Thought Consequences	
Challenge your Initial Thought	
Negative Thinking	
Background	
Alternative Thinking	
Positive Belief and Affirmation	
Action Plan	
Improvement	

Dr's Notes: _____

_____

Name: _____ Date: _____ Sign: _____

© 2019 Portia Cruise. *Cognitive Behavioral Therapy Worksheets.* Copyrighted Material

Worksheets for Cognitive Behavioral Therapy

Date: ___/___/____

Situation	
Initial Thought	
Thought Consequences	
Challenge your Initial Thought	
Negative Thinking	
Background	
Alternative Thinking	
Positive Belief and Affirmation	
Action Plan	
Improvement	

Dr's Notes: _____

_____

Name: _____ Date: _____ Sign: _____

© 2019 Portia Cruise. *Cognitive Behavioral Therapy Worksheets.* Copyrighted Material

Worksheets for Cognitive Behavioral Therapy

Date: ____/____/_____

Situation	
Initial Thought	
Thought Consequences	
Challenge your Initial Thought	
Negative Thinking	
Background	
Alternative Thinking	
Positive Belief and Affirmation	
Action Plan	
Improvement	

Dr's Notes: _____

_____

Name: _____ Date: _____ Sign: _____

© 2019 Portia Cruise. *Cognitive Behavioral Therapy Worksheets.* **Copyrighted Material**

Worksheets for Cognitive Behavioral Therapy

Date: ____/____/_____

Situation	
Initial Thought	
Thought Consequences	
Challenge your Initial Thought	
Negative Thinking	
Background	
Alternative Thinking	
Positive Belief and Affirmation	
Action Plan	
Improvement	

Dr's Notes: _____

_____

Name: _____ Date: _____ Sign: _____

© 2019 Portia Cruise. *Cognitive Behavioral Therapy Worksheets.* **Copyrighted Material**

Worksheets for Cognitive Behavioral Therapy

Date: ____/____/_____

Situation	
Initial Thought	
Thought Consequences	
Challenge your Initial Thought	
Negative Thinking	
Background	
Alternative Thinking	
Positive Belief and Affirmation	
Action Plan	
Improvement	

Dr's Notes: _____

_____

Name: _____ Date: _____ Sign: _____

© 2019 Portia Cruise. *Cognitive Behavioral Therapy Worksheets.* **Copyrighted Material**

Worksheets for Cognitive Behavioral Therapy

Date: ____/____/_____

Situation	
Initial Thought	
Thought Consequences	
Challenge your Initial Thought	
Negative Thinking	
Background	
Alternative Thinking	
Positive Belief and Affirmation	
Action Plan	
Improvement	

Dr's Notes: _____

_____

Name: _____ Date: _____ Sign: _____

© 2019 Portia Cruise. *Cognitive Behavioral Therapy Worksheets.* **Copyrighted Material**

Worksheets for Cognitive Behavioral Therapy

Date: ____/____/_____

Situation	
Initial Thought	
Thought Consequences	
Challenge your Initial Thought	
Negative Thinking	
Background	
Alternative Thinking	
Positive Belief and Affirmation	
Action Plan	
Improvement	

Dr's Notes: _____

_____

Name: _____ Date: _____ Sign: _____

© 2019 Portia Cruise. *Cognitive Behavioral Therapy Worksheets.* Copyrighted Material

Worksheets for Cognitive Behavioral Therapy

Date: ____/____/_____

Situation	
Initial Thought	
Thought Consequences	
Challenge your Initial Thought	
Negative Thinking	
Background	
Alternative Thinking	
Positive Belief and Affirmation	
Action Plan	
Improvement	

Dr's Notes: _____

_____

Name: _____ Date: _____ Sign: _____

© 2019 Portia Cruise. *Cognitive Behavioral Therapy Worksheets.* **Copyrighted Material**

Worksheets for Cognitive Behavioral Therapy

Date: ___/___/_____

Situation	
Initial Thought	
Thought Consequences	
Challenge your Initial Thought	
Negative Thinking	
Background	
Alternative Thinking	
Positive Belief and Affirmation	
Action Plan	
Improvement	

Dr's Notes: _____

_____

Name: _____ Date: _____ Sign: _____

© 2019 Portia Cruise. *Cognitive Behavioral Therapy Worksheets.* **Copyrighted Material**

Worksheets for Cognitive Behavioral Therapy

Date: ___/___/_____

Situation	
Initial Thought	
Thought Consequences	
Challenge your Initial Thought	
Negative Thinking	
Background	
Alternative Thinking	
Positive Belief and Affirmation	
Action Plan	
Improvement	

Dr's Notes: _____

_____

Name: _____ Date: _____ Sign: _____

© 2019 Portia Cruise. *Cognitive Behavioral Therapy Worksheets.* Copyrighted Material

Worksheets for Cognitive Behavioral Therapy

Date: ___/___/_____

Situation	
Initial Thought	
Thought Consequences	
Challenge your Initial Thought	
Negative Thinking	
Background	
Alternative Thinking	
Positive Belief and Affirmation	
Action Plan	
Improvement	

Dr's Notes: _____

_____

Name: _____ Date: _____ Sign: _____

© 2019 Portia Cruise. *Cognitive Behavioral Therapy Worksheets.* **Copyrighted Material**

Worksheets for Cognitive Behavioral Therapy

Date: ____/____/_____

Situation	
Initial Thought	
Thought Consequences	
Challenge your Initial Thought	
Negative Thinking	
Background	
Alternative Thinking	
Positive Belief and Affirmation	
Action Plan	
Improvement	

Dr's Notes: _____

_____

Name: _____ Date: _____ Sign: _____

© 2019 Portia Cruise. *Cognitive Behavioral Therapy Worksheets.* **Copyrighted Material**

Worksheets for Cognitive Behavioral Therapy

Date: ___/___/_____

Situation	
Initial Thought	
Thought Consequences	
Challenge your Initial Thought	
Negative Thinking	
Background	
Alternative Thinking	
Positive Belief and Affirmation	
Action Plan	
Improvement	

Dr's Notes: _____

_____

Name: _____ Date: _____ Sign: _____

© 2019 Portia Cruise. *Cognitive Behavioral Therapy Worksheets.* **Copyrighted Material**

Worksheets for Cognitive Behavioral Therapy

Date: ____/____/_____

Situation	
Initial Thought	
Thought Consequences	
Challenge your Initial Thought	
Negative Thinking	
Background	
Alternative Thinking	
Positive Belief and Affirmation	
Action Plan	
Improvement	

Dr's Notes: _____

_____

Name: _____ Date: _____ Sign: _____

© 2019 Portia Cruise. *Cognitive Behavioral Therapy Worksheets.* **Copyrighted Material**

Worksheets for Cognitive Behavioral Therapy

Date: ____/____/_____

Situation	
Initial Thought	
Thought Consequences	
Challenge your Initial Thought	
Negative Thinking	
Background	
Alternative Thinking	
Positive Belief and Affirmation	
Action Plan	
Improvement	

Dr's Notes: _____

_____

Name: _____ Date: _____ Sign: _____

© 2019 Portia Cruise. *Cognitive Behavioral Therapy Worksheets.* **Copyrighted Material**

Worksheets for Cognitive Behavioral Therapy

Date: ___/___/_____

Situation	
Initial Thought	
Thought Consequences	
Challenge your Initial Thought	
Negative Thinking	
Background	
Alternative Thinking	
Positive Belief and Affirmation	
Action Plan	
Improvement	

Dr's Notes: _____

_____

Name: _____ Date: _____ Sign: _____

© 2019 Portia Cruise. *Cognitive Behavioral Therapy Worksheets.* Copyrighted Material

Worksheets for Cognitive Behavioral Therapy

Date: ___/___/_____

Situation	
Initial Thought	
Thought Consequences	
Challenge your Initial Thought	
Negative Thinking	
Background	
Alternative Thinking	
Positive Belief and Affirmation	
Action Plan	
Improvement	

Dr's Notes: _____

_____

Name: _____ Date: _____ Sign: _____

© 2019 Portia Cruise. *Cognitive Behavioral Therapy Worksheets.* Copyrighted Material

Worksheets for Cognitive Behavioral Therapy

Date: ____/____/_____

Situation	
Initial Thought	
Thought Consequences	
Challenge your Initial Thought	
Negative Thinking	
Background	
Alternative Thinking	
Positive Belief and Affirmation	
Action Plan	
Improvement	

Dr's Notes: _____

_____

Name: _____ Date: _____ Sign: _____

© 2019 Portia Cruise. *Cognitive Behavioral Therapy Worksheets.* **Copyrighted Material**

Worksheets for Cognitive Behavioral Therapy

Date: ___/___/_____

Situation	
Initial Thought	
Thought Consequences	
Challenge your Initial Thought	
Negative Thinking	
Background	
Alternative Thinking	
Positive Belief and Affirmation	
Action Plan	
Improvement	

Dr's Notes: _____

_____

Name: _____ Date: _____ Sign: _____

© 2019 Portia Cruise. *Cognitive Behavioral Therapy Worksheets.* **Copyrighted Material**

Worksheets for Cognitive Behavioral Therapy

Date: ____/____/_____

Situation	
Initial Thought	
Thought Consequences	
Challenge your Initial Thought	
Negative Thinking	
Background	
Alternative Thinking	
Positive Belief and Affirmation	
Action Plan	
Improvement	

Dr's Notes: _____

_____

Name: _____ Date: _____ Sign: _____

© 2019 Portia Cruise. *Cognitive Behavioral Therapy Worksheets.* **Copyrighted Material**

Worksheets for Cognitive Behavioral Therapy

Date: ___/___/_____

Situation	
Initial Thought	
Thought Consequences	
Challenge your Initial Thought	
Negative Thinking	
Background	
Alternative Thinking	
Positive Belief and Affirmation	
Action Plan	
Improvement	

Dr's Notes: _____

_____

Name: _____ Date: _____ Sign: _____

© 2019 Portia Cruise. *Cognitive Behavioral Therapy Worksheets.* Copyrighted Material

Worksheets for Cognitive Behavioral Therapy

Date: ___/___/_____

Situation	
Initial Thought	
Thought Consequences	
Challenge your Initial Thought	
Negative Thinking	
Background	
Alternative Thinking	
Positive Belief and Affirmation	
Action Plan	
Improvement	

Dr's Notes: _____

_____

Name: _____   Date: _____   Sign: _____

© 2019 Portia Cruise. *Cognitive Behavioral Therapy Worksheets.* **Copyrighted Material**

Worksheets for Cognitive Behavioral Therapy

Date: ____/____/_____

Situation	
Initial Thought	
Thought Consequences	
Challenge your Initial Thought	
Negative Thinking	
Background	
Alternative Thinking	
Positive Belief and Affirmation	
Action Plan	
Improvement	

Dr's Notes: _____

_____

Name: _____   Date: _____   Sign: _____

© 2019 Portia Cruise. *Cognitive Behavioral Therapy Worksheets.* Copyrighted Material

Worksheets for Cognitive Behavioral Therapy

Date: ___/___/_____

Situation	
Initial Thought	
Thought Consequences	
Challenge your Initial Thought	
Negative Thinking	
Background	
Alternative Thinking	
Positive Belief and Affirmation	
Action Plan	
Improvement	

Dr's Notes: _____

_____

Name: _____ Date: _____ Sign: _____

© 2019 Portia Cruise. *Cognitive Behavioral Therapy Worksheets.* **Copyrighted Material**

Worksheets for Cognitive Behavioral Therapy

Date: ___/___/_____

Situation	
Initial Thought	
Thought Consequences	
Challenge your Initial Thought	
Negative Thinking	
Background	
Alternative Thinking	
Positive Belief and Affirmation	
Action Plan	
Improvement	

Dr's Notes: _____

_____

Name: _____ Date: _____ Sign: _____

© 2019 Portia Cruise. *Cognitive Behavioral Therapy Worksheets.* **Copyrighted Material**

Worksheets for Cognitive Behavioral Therapy

Date: ____/____/_____

Situation	
Initial Thought	
Thought Consequences	
Challenge your Initial Thought	
Negative Thinking	
Background	
Alternative Thinking	
Positive Belief and Affirmation	
Action Plan	
Improvement	

Dr's Notes: _____

_____

Name: _____ Date: _____ Sign: _____

© 2019 Portia Cruise. *Cognitive Behavioral Therapy Worksheets.* **Copyrighted Material**

Worksheets for Cognitive Behavioral Therapy

Date: ___/___/_____

Situation	
Initial Thought	
Thought Consequences	
Challenge your Initial Thought	
Negative Thinking	
Background	
Alternative Thinking	
Positive Belief and Affirmation	
Action Plan	
Improvement	

Dr's Notes: _____

_____

Name: _____ Date: _____ Sign: _____

© 2019 Portia Cruise. *Cognitive Behavioral Therapy Worksheets.* Copyrighted Material

Worksheets for Cognitive Behavioral Therapy

Date: ____/____/_____

Situation	
Initial Thought	
Thought Consequences	
Challenge your Initial Thought	
Negative Thinking	
Background	
Alternative Thinking	
Positive Belief and Affirmation	
Action Plan	
Improvement	

Dr's Notes: _____

_____

Name: _____ Date: _____ Sign: _____

© 2019 Portia Cruise. *Cognitive Behavioral Therapy Worksheets.* **Copyrighted Material**

Worksheets for Cognitive Behavioral Therapy

Date: ___/___/_____

Situation	
Initial Thought	
Thought Consequences	
Challenge your Initial Thought	
Negative Thinking	
Background	
Alternative Thinking	
Positive Belief and Affirmation	
Action Plan	
Improvement	

Dr's Notes: _____

_____

Name: _____ Date: _____ Sign: _____

© 2019 Portia Cruise. *Cognitive Behavioral Therapy Worksheets.* **Copyrighted Material**

Worksheets for Cognitive Behavioral Therapy

Date: ____/____/_____

Situation	
Initial Thought	
Thought Consequences	
Challenge your Initial Thought	
Negative Thinking	
Background	
Alternative Thinking	
Positive Belief and Affirmation	
Action Plan	
Improvement	

Dr's Notes: _____

_____

Name: _____ Date: _____ Sign: _____

© 2019 Portia Cruise. *Cognitive Behavioral Therapy Worksheets.* Copyrighted Material

Worksheets for Cognitive Behavioral Therapy

Date: ____/____/_____

Situation	
Initial Thought	
Thought Consequences	
Challenge your Initial Thought	
Negative Thinking	
Background	
Alternative Thinking	
Positive Belief and Affirmation	
Action Plan	
Improvement	

Dr's Notes: _____

_____

Name: _____ Date: _____ Sign: _____

© 2019 Portia Cruise. *Cognitive Behavioral Therapy Worksheets.* **Copyrighted Material**

Worksheets for Cognitive Behavioral Therapy

Date: ___/___/_____

Situation	
Initial Thought	
Thought Consequences	
Challenge your Initial Thought	
Negative Thinking	
Background	
Alternative Thinking	
Positive Belief and Affirmation	
Action Plan	
Improvement	

Dr's Notes: _____

_____

Name: _____ Date: _____ Sign: _____

© 2019 Portia Cruise. *Cognitive Behavioral Therapy Worksheets.* **Copyrighted Material**

Worksheets for Cognitive Behavioral Therapy

Date: ___/___/_____

Situation	
Initial Thought	
Thought Consequences	
Challenge your Initial Thought	
Negative Thinking	
Background	
Alternative Thinking	
Positive Belief and Affirmation	
Action Plan	
Improvement	

Dr's Notes: _____

_____

Name: _____ Date: _____ Sign: _____

© 2019 Portia Cruise. *Cognitive Behavioral Therapy Worksheets.* Copyrighted Material

Worksheets for Cognitive Behavioral Therapy

Date: ____/____/_____

Situation	
Initial Thought	
Thought Consequences	
Challenge your Initial Thought	
Negative Thinking	
Background	
Alternative Thinking	
Positive Belief and Affirmation	
Action Plan	
Improvement	

Dr's Notes: _____

_____

Name: _____ Date: _____ Sign: _____

© 2019 Portia Cruise. *Cognitive Behavioral Therapy Worksheets.* **Copyrighted Material**

Worksheets for Cognitive Behavioral Therapy

Date: ____/____/_____

Situation	
Initial Thought	
Thought Consequences	
Challenge your Initial Thought	
Negative Thinking	
Background	
Alternative Thinking	
Positive Belief and Affirmation	
Action Plan	
Improvement	

Dr's Notes: _____

_____

Name: _____ Date: _____ Sign: _____

© 2019 Portia Cruise. *Cognitive Behavioral Therapy Worksheets.* **Copyrighted Material**

Worksheets for Cognitive Behavioral Therapy

Date: ___/___/_____

Situation	
Initial Thought	
Thought Consequences	
Challenge your Initial Thought	
Negative Thinking	
Background	
Alternative Thinking	
Positive Belief and Affirmation	
Action Plan	
Improvement	

Dr's Notes: _____

_____

Name: _____ Date: _____ Sign: _____

© 2019 Portia Cruise. *Cognitive Behavioral Therapy Worksheets.* Copyrighted Material

Worksheets for Cognitive Behavioral Therapy

Date: ___/___/____

Situation	
Initial Thought	
Thought Consequences	
Challenge your Initial Thought	
Negative Thinking	
Background	
Alternative Thinking	
Positive Belief and Affirmation	
Action Plan	
Improvement	

Dr's Notes: _____

Name: _____ Date: _____ Sign: _____

© 2019 Portia Cruise. *Cognitive Behavioral Therapy Worksheets.* **Copyrighted Material**

Worksheets for Cognitive Behavioral Therapy

Date: ____/____/_____

Situation	
Initial Thought	
Thought Consequences	
Challenge your Initial Thought	
Negative Thinking	
Background	
Alternative Thinking	
Positive Belief and Affirmation	
Action Plan	
Improvement	

Dr's Notes: _____

_____

Name: _____ Date: _____ Sign: _____

© 2019 Portia Cruise. *Cognitive Behavioral Therapy Worksheets.* Copyrighted Material

Worksheets for Cognitive Behavioral Therapy

Date: ___/___/_____

Situation	
Initial Thought	
Thought Consequences	
Challenge your Initial Thought	
Negative Thinking	
Background	
Alternative Thinking	
Positive Belief and Affirmation	
Action Plan	
Improvement	

Dr's Notes: _____

_____

Name: _____ Date: _____ Sign: _____

© 2019 Portia Cruise. *Cognitive Behavioral Therapy Worksheets.* Copyrighted Material

Worksheets for Cognitive Behavioral Therapy

Date: ____/____/_____

Situation	
Initial Thought	
Thought Consequences	
Challenge your Initial Thought	
Negative Thinking	
Background	
Alternative Thinking	
Positive Belief and Affirmation	
Action Plan	
Improvement	

Dr's Notes: _____

_____

Name: _____ Date: _____ Sign: _____

© 2019 Portia Cruise. *Cognitive Behavioral Therapy Worksheets.* **Copyrighted Material**

Worksheets for Cognitive Behavioral Therapy

Date: ____/____/_____

Situation	
Initial Thought	
Thought Consequences	
Challenge your Initial Thought	
Negative Thinking	
Background	
Alternative Thinking	
Positive Belief and Affirmation	
Action Plan	
Improvement	

Dr's Notes: _____

_____

Name: _____ Date: _____ Sign: _____

© 2019 Portia Cruise. *Cognitive Behavioral Therapy Worksheets.* **Copyrighted Material**

Worksheets for Cognitive Behavioral Therapy

Date: ____/____/_____

Situation	
Initial Thought	
Thought Consequences	
Challenge your Initial Thought	
Negative Thinking	
Background	
Alternative Thinking	
Positive Belief and Affirmation	
Action Plan	
Improvement	

Dr's Notes: _____

_____

Name: _____ Date: _____ Sign: _____

© 2019 Portia Cruise. *Cognitive Behavioral Therapy Worksheets.* Copyrighted Material

Worksheets for Cognitive Behavioral Therapy

Date: ___/___/_____

Situation	
Initial Thought	
Thought Consequences	
Challenge your Initial Thought	
Negative Thinking	
Background	
Alternative Thinking	
Positive Belief and Affirmation	
Action Plan	
Improvement	

Dr's Notes: _____

_____

Name: _____ Date: _____ Sign: _____

© 2019 Portia Cruise. *Cognitive Behavioral Therapy Worksheets.* Copyrighted Material

Worksheets for Cognitive Behavioral Therapy

Date: ____/____/_____

Situation	
Initial Thought	
Thought Consequences	
Challenge your Initial Thought	
Negative Thinking	
Background	
Alternative Thinking	
Positive Belief and Affirmation	
Action Plan	
Improvement	

Dr's Notes: _____

_____

Name: _____ Date: _____ Sign: _____

© 2019 Portia Cruise. *Cognitive Behavioral Therapy Worksheets.* **Copyrighted Material**

Worksheets for Cognitive Behavioral Therapy

Date: ____/____/_____

Situation	
Initial Thought	
Thought Consequences	
Challenge your Initial Thought	
Negative Thinking	
Background	
Alternative Thinking	
Positive Belief and Affirmation	
Action Plan	
Improvement	

Dr's Notes: _____

_____

Name: _____ Date: _____ Sign: _____

© 2019 Portia Cruise. *Cognitive Behavioral Therapy Worksheets.* **Copyrighted Material**

Worksheets for Cognitive Behavioral Therapy

Date: ____/____/_____

Situation	
Initial Thought	
Thought Consequences	
Challenge your Initial Thought	
Negative Thinking	
Background	
Alternative Thinking	
Positive Belief and Affirmation	
Action Plan	
Improvement	

Dr's Notes: _____

_____

Name: _____ Date: _____ Sign: _____

© 2019 Portia Cruise. *Cognitive Behavioral Therapy Worksheets.* **Copyrighted Material**

Worksheets for Cognitive Behavioral Therapy

Date: ____/____/_____

Situation	
Initial Thought	
Thought Consequences	
Challenge your Initial Thought	
Negative Thinking	
Background	
Alternative Thinking	
Positive Belief and Affirmation	
Action Plan	
Improvement	

Dr's Notes: _____

_____

Name: _____ Date: _____ Sign: _____

© 2019 Portia Cruise. *Cognitive Behavioral Therapy Worksheets.* **Copyrighted Material**

Worksheets for Cognitive Behavioral Therapy

Date: ____/____/_____

Situation	
Initial Thought	
Thought Consequences	
Challenge your Initial Thought	
Negative Thinking	
Background	
Alternative Thinking	
Positive Belief and Affirmation	
Action Plan	
Improvement	

Dr's Notes: _____

_____

Name: _____ Date: _____ Sign: _____

© 2019 Portia Cruise. *Cognitive Behavioral Therapy Worksheets.* **Copyrighted Material**

Worksheets for Cognitive Behavioral Therapy

Date: ____/____/_____

Situation	
Initial Thought	
Thought Consequences	
Challenge your Initial Thought	
Negative Thinking	
Background	
Alternative Thinking	
Positive Belief and Affirmation	
Action Plan	
Improvement	

Dr's Notes: _____

_____

Name: _____ Date: _____ Sign: _____

© 2019 Portia Cruise. *Cognitive Behavioral Therapy Worksheets.* **Copyrighted Material**

Worksheets for Cognitive Behavioral Therapy

Date: ___/___/_____

Situation	
Initial Thought	
Thought Consequences	
Challenge your Initial Thought	
Negative Thinking	
Background	
Alternative Thinking	
Positive Belief and Affirmation	
Action Plan	
Improvement	

Dr's Notes: _____

_____

Name: _____ Date: _____ Sign: _____

© 2019 Portia Cruise. *Cognitive Behavioral Therapy Worksheets.* **Copyrighted Material**

Worksheets for Cognitive Behavioral Therapy

Date: ____/____/_____

Situation	
Initial Thought	
Thought Consequences	
Challenge your Initial Thought	
Negative Thinking	
Background	
Alternative Thinking	
Positive Belief and Affirmation	
Action Plan	
Improvement	

Dr's Notes: _____

_____

Name: _____   Date: _____   Sign: _____

© 2019 Portia Cruise. *Cognitive Behavioral Therapy Worksheets.* Copyrighted Material

Worksheets for Cognitive Behavioral Therapy

Date: ____/____/_____

Situation	
Initial Thought	
Thought Consequences	
Challenge your Initial Thought	
Negative Thinking	
Background	
Alternative Thinking	
Positive Belief and Affirmation	
Action Plan	
Improvement	

Dr's Notes: _____

_____

Name: _____ Date: _____ Sign: _____

© 2019 Portia Cruise. *Cognitive Behavioral Therapy Worksheets.* **Copyrighted Material**

Worksheets for Cognitive Behavioral Therapy

Date: ____/____/_____

Situation	
Initial Thought	
Thought Consequences	
Challenge your Initial Thought	
Negative Thinking	
Background	
Alternative Thinking	
Positive Belief and Affirmation	
Action Plan	
Improvement	

Dr's Notes: _____

_____

Name: _____   Date: _____   Sign: _____

© 2019 Portia Cruise. *Cognitive Behavioral Therapy Worksheets.* **Copyrighted Material**

Worksheets for Cognitive Behavioral Therapy

Date: ____/____/_____

Situation	
Initial Thought	
Thought Consequences	
Challenge your Initial Thought	
Negative Thinking	
Background	
Alternative Thinking	
Positive Belief and Affirmation	
Action Plan	
Improvement	

Dr's Notes: _____

_____

Name: _____   Date: _____   Sign: _____

© 2019 Portia Cruise. *Cognitive Behavioral Therapy Worksheets.* **Copyrighted Material**

Worksheets for Cognitive Behavioral Therapy

Date: ___/___/_____

Situation	
Initial Thought	
Thought Consequences	
Challenge your Initial Thought	
Negative Thinking	
Background	
Alternative Thinking	
Positive Belief and Affirmation	
Action Plan	
Improvement	

Dr's Notes: _____

_____

Name: _____ Date: _____ Sign: _____

© 2019 Portia Cruise. *Cognitive Behavioral Therapy Worksheets.* Copyrighted Material

Worksheets for Cognitive Behavioral Therapy

Date: ___/___/_____

Situation	
Initial Thought	
Thought Consequences	
Challenge your Initial Thought	
Negative Thinking	
Background	
Alternative Thinking	
Positive Belief and Affirmation	
Action Plan	
Improvement	

Dr's Notes: _____

_____

Name: _____ Date: _____ Sign: _____

© 2019 Portia Cruise. *Cognitive Behavioral Therapy Worksheets.* Copyrighted Material

Worksheets for Cognitive Behavioral Therapy

Date: ___/___/_____

Situation	
Initial Thought	
Thought Consequences	
Challenge your Initial Thought	
Negative Thinking	
Background	
Alternative Thinking	
Positive Belief and Affirmation	
Action Plan	
Improvement	

Dr's Notes: _____

_____

Name: _____ Date: _____ Sign: _____

© 2019 Portia Cruise. *Cognitive Behavioral Therapy Worksheets.* **Copyrighted Material**

Worksheets for Cognitive Behavioral Therapy

Date: ___/___/_____

Situation	
Initial Thought	
Thought Consequences	
Challenge your Initial Thought	
Negative Thinking	
Background	
Alternative Thinking	
Positive Belief and Affirmation	
Action Plan	
Improvement	

Dr's Notes: _____

_____

Name: _____ Date: _____ Sign: _____

© 2019 Portia Cruise. *Cognitive Behavioral Therapy Worksheets.* Copyrighted Material

Worksheets for Cognitive Behavioral Therapy

Date: ___/___/_____

Situation	
Initial Thought	
Thought Consequences	
Challenge your Initial Thought	
Negative Thinking	
Background	
Alternative Thinking	
Positive Belief and Affirmation	
Action Plan	
Improvement	

Dr's Notes: _____

_____

Name: _____ Date: _____ Sign: _____

© 2019 Portia Cruise. *Cognitive Behavioral Therapy Worksheets.* **Copyrighted Material**

Worksheets for Cognitive Behavioral Therapy

Date: ____/____/_____

Situation	
Initial Thought	
Thought Consequences	
Challenge your Initial Thought	
Negative Thinking	
Background	
Alternative Thinking	
Positive Belief and Affirmation	
Action Plan	
Improvement	

Dr's Notes: _____

_____

Name: _____ Date: _____ Sign: _____

© 2019 Portia Cruise. *Cognitive Behavioral Therapy Worksheets.* Copyrighted Material

Worksheets for Cognitive Behavioral Therapy

Date: ___/___/_____

Situation	
Initial Thought	
Thought Consequences	
Challenge your Initial Thought	
Negative Thinking	
Background	
Alternative Thinking	
Positive Belief and Affirmation	
Action Plan	
Improvement	

Dr's Notes: _____

_____

Name: _____ Date: _____ Sign: _____

© 2019 Portia Cruise. *Cognitive Behavioral Therapy Worksheets.* Copyrighted Material

Worksheets for Cognitive Behavioral Therapy

Date: ___/___/_____

Situation	
Initial Thought	
Thought Consequences	
Challenge your Initial Thought	
Negative Thinking	
Background	
Alternative Thinking	
Positive Belief and Affirmation	
Action Plan	
Improvement	

Dr's Notes: _____

_____

Name: _____ Date: _____ Sign: _____

© 2019 Portia Cruise. *Cognitive Behavioral Therapy Worksheets.* **Copyrighted Material**

Worksheets for Cognitive Behavioral Therapy

Date: ___/___/_____

Situation	
Initial Thought	
Thought Consequences	
Challenge your Initial Thought	
Negative Thinking	
Background	
Alternative Thinking	
Positive Belief and Affirmation	
Action Plan	
Improvement	

Dr's Notes: _____

_____

Name: _____ Date: _____ Sign: _____

© 2019 Portia Cruise. *Cognitive Behavioral Therapy Worksheets.* Copyrighted Material

Worksheets for Cognitive Behavioral Therapy

Date: ___/___/_____

Situation	
Initial Thought	
Thought Consequences	
Challenge your Initial Thought	
Negative Thinking	
Background	
Alternative Thinking	
Positive Belief and Affirmation	
Action Plan	
Improvement	

Dr's Notes: _____

_____

Name: _____ Date: _____ Sign: _____

© 2019 Portia Cruise. *Cognitive Behavioral Therapy Worksheets.* **Copyrighted Material**

Worksheets for Cognitive Behavioral Therapy

Date: ___/___/_____

Situation	
Initial Thought	
Thought Consequences	
Challenge your Initial Thought	
Negative Thinking	
Background	
Alternative Thinking	
Positive Belief and Affirmation	
Action Plan	
Improvement	

Dr's Notes: _____

_____

Name: _____ Date: _____ Sign: _____

© 2019 Portia Cruise. *Cognitive Behavioral Therapy Worksheets.* **Copyrighted Material**

Worksheets for Cognitive Behavioral Therapy

Date: ___/___/_____

Situation	
Initial Thought	
Thought Consequences	
Challenge your Initial Thought	
Negative Thinking	
Background	
Alternative Thinking	
Positive Belief and Affirmation	
Action Plan	
Improvement	

Dr's Notes: _____

_____

Name: _____ Date: _____ Sign: _____

© 2019 Portia Cruise. *Cognitive Behavioral Therapy Worksheets.* **Copyrighted Material**

Worksheets for Cognitive Behavioral Therapy

Date: ___/___/_____

Situation	
Initial Thought	
Thought Consequences	
Challenge your Initial Thought	
Negative Thinking	
Background	
Alternative Thinking	
Positive Belief and Affirmation	
Action Plan	
Improvement	

Dr's Notes: _____

_____

Name: _____ Date: _____ Sign: _____

Worksheets for Cognitive Behavioral Therapy

Date: ___/___/_____

Situation	
Initial Thought	
Thought Consequences	
Challenge your Initial Thought	
Negative Thinking	
Background	
Alternative Thinking	
Positive Belief and Affirmation	
Action Plan	
Improvement	

Dr's Notes: _____

_____

Name: _____ Date: _____ Sign: _____

© 2019 Portia Cruise. *Cognitive Behavioral Therapy Worksheets.* **Copyrighted Material**

Worksheets for Cognitive Behavioral Therapy

Date: ___/___/_____

Situation	
Initial Thought	
Thought Consequences	
Challenge your Initial Thought	
Negative Thinking	
Background	
Alternative Thinking	
Positive Belief and Affirmation	
Action Plan	
Improvement	

Dr's Notes: _____

_____

Name: _____ Date: _____ Sign: _____

© 2019 Portia Cruise. *Cognitive Behavioral Therapy Worksheets.* Copyrighted Material

Worksheets for Cognitive Behavioral Therapy

Date: ___/___/_____

Situation	
Initial Thought	
Thought Consequences	
Challenge your Initial Thought	
Negative Thinking	
Background	
Alternative Thinking	
Positive Belief and Affirmation	
Action Plan	
Improvement	

Dr's Notes: _____

_____

Name: _____ Date: _____ Sign: _____

© 2019 Portia Cruise. *Cognitive Behavioral Therapy Worksheets.* **Copyrighted Material**

Worksheets for Cognitive Behavioral Therapy

Date: ___/___/_____

Situation	
Initial Thought	
Thought Consequences	
Challenge your Initial Thought	
Negative Thinking	
Background	
Alternative Thinking	
Positive Belief and Affirmation	
Action Plan	
Improvement	

Dr's Notes: _____

_____

Name: _____ Date: _____ Sign: _____

© 2019 Portia Cruise. *Cognitive Behavioral Therapy Worksheets.* **Copyrighted Material**

Worksheets for Cognitive Behavioral Therapy

Date: ____/____/_____

Situation	
Initial Thought	
Thought Consequences	
Challenge your Initial Thought	
Negative Thinking	
Background	
Alternative Thinking	
Positive Belief and Affirmation	
Action Plan	
Improvement	

Dr's Notes: _____

_____

Name: _____ Date: _____ Sign: _____

© 2019 Portia Cruise. *Cognitive Behavioral Therapy Worksheets.* Copyrighted Material

Worksheets for Cognitive Behavioral Therapy

Date: ___/___/_____

Situation	
Initial Thought	
Thought Consequences	
Challenge your Initial Thought	
Negative Thinking	
Background	
Alternative Thinking	
Positive Belief and Affirmation	
Action Plan	
Improvement	

Dr's Notes: _____

_____

Name: _____ Date: _____ Sign: _____

© 2019 Portia Cruise. *Cognitive Behavioral Therapy Worksheets.* **Copyrighted Material**

Worksheets for Cognitive Behavioral Therapy

Date: ___/___/_____

Situation	
Initial Thought	
Thought Consequences	
Challenge your Initial Thought	
Negative Thinking	
Background	
Alternative Thinking	
Positive Belief and Affirmation	
Action Plan	
Improvement	

Dr's Notes: _____

_____

Name: _____ Date: _____ Sign: _____

© 2019 Portia Cruise. *Cognitive Behavioral Therapy Worksheets.* **Copyrighted Material**

Worksheets for Cognitive Behavioral Therapy

Date: ___/___/_____

Situation	
Initial Thought	
Thought Consequences	
Challenge your Initial Thought	
Negative Thinking	
Background	
Alternative Thinking	
Positive Belief and Affirmation	
Action Plan	
Improvement	

Dr's Notes: _____

_____

Name: _____ Date: _____ Sign: _____

© 2019 Portia Cruise. *Cognitive Behavioral Therapy Worksheets.* Copyrighted Material

Note

Note

Note

Note

www.ingramcontent.com/pod-product-compliance
Lightning Source LLC
Chambersburg PA
CBHW070654220526
45466CB00001B/432